THE EXTREME METABOLIC CONFUSION DIET FOR WOMEN

Discover the path to optimal health, weight loss, and hormonal balance through proven strategies, effective exercises, a 30-day meal plan, and delightful recipes and food lists.

Vincent John Walker

DISCLAIMER

Table of Contents

INTRODUCTION

Women are often confronted with a confusing variety of food trends in their pursuit of maximum health and wellbeing, many of which claim to be the secret to their ideal state of physical and mental wellbeing. Women have been exposed to a wide range of dietary regimens, from the low-fat craze of the 1990s to the more recent wave of interest in ketogenic diets. The Metabolic Confusion Diet, however, stands out amid this clamor because it has the potential to change how women interact with their bodies and metabolisms.

Think about a diet that honors the complex and distinctive qualities of the female body rather than confining you to strict, one-size-fits-all guidelines. Imagine a way of eating that, in addition to honoring your body's hormonal needs, really uses its powerful effect to transform your life. This is the core of the groundbreaking Metabolic Confusion Diet, created especially for the fascinating variety of women.

Our trip starts with a basic comprehension of Metabolic Confusion, the idea at the core of this revolutionary technique.

Understanding Metabolic Perplexity

Metabolic Confusion is a paradigm change in our understanding of and interactions with our metabolism, not simply another fad diet fad. It acknowledges that women's bodies are complex, dynamic systems that are impacted by a wide range of circumstances rather than static entities. Every woman's metabolism is a symphony of complexity, influenced by everything from hormones that march to their rhythm to the sway of age and genetic imprints.

Fundamentally, Metabolic Confusion does not seek to oversimplify this complexity; rather, it embraces it. It recognizes that a woman's metabolic requirements are not set in stone, that diets that are too strict may leave people feeling disappointed and frustrated, and that what works today might not work tomorrow.

Instead of fighting against our metabolism, Metabolic Confusion encourages us to work with it. It entails strategically varying the meals we eat when we eat, and even what kinds of foods we eat to keep our bodies guessing, avoid adaptation, and guarantee continuous improvement. It releases the powerful force of hormonal balance to promote weight reduction, long-lasting energy, and general health.

As we explore the world of the Metabolic Confusion Diet for Women in more detail, you will discover how this strategy can be adjusted to meet your specific needs and help you achieve your goals for fitness and health in a way that feels natural and long-lasting. You will learn the science behind Metabolic Confusion and how it helps women overcome the typical obstacles they face on their path to radiant health.

So let's go out on this life-changing journey together, one that will completely change the way you understand nutrition and metabolism and give you the tools you need to take charge of your health and become the strong, self-assured woman you were meant to be. Greetings from the land of Metabolic Confusion, where the true potential of your body waits to be discovered.

WOMEN'S PARTICULAR METABOLIC CHALLENGES

The complexity of the human body is fascinating, and when it comes to metabolism, women's physiology provides its own set of unique issues and concerns. Understanding these unique characteristics is essential for building effective and long-term dietary and lifestyle decisions. Let's take a look at the complicated terrain of women's metabolic disorders.

Hormone fluctuations

Managing the Ebb and Flow of Women's Hormones

Hormonal fluctuations are an inherent part of a woman's life, affecting not just her reproductive system but also her metabolism, temperament, and general health. These changes are a natural and difficult component of the female experience, but they also provide new health and lifestyle management challenges and opportunities. Let's take a look at hormone shifts and how they affect women's lives.

Hormones During the Menstrual Cycle and the Monthly Dance

The menstrual cycle is the pulse of female hormonal fluctuations. Individual variances occur, but they normally last around 28 days. The following hormones play critical roles in organizing this complex dance:

- **Estrogen:** This hormone rises throughout the first half of the menstrual cycle (the follicular phase). It increases energy and well-being by thickening the uterine lining in preparation for a pregnancy.

- **Progesterone:** Progesterone takes center stage in the second half of the cycle (the luteal phase). It aids in the retention of the uterine lining and modulates mood and appetite.

- **Luteinizing Hormone (LH) and Follicle-Stimulating Hormone (FSH):** These hormones rise and fall to stimulate ovarian follicle development and ovulation.

During the cycle, these hormonal oscillations may induce variations in metabolic rate, energy levels, and even food appetites. Understanding these hormonal fluctuations may help women make sensible nutritional choices throughout their menstrual cycle, with a focus on nutrient-rich meals to boost energy levels and emotional stability.

Pregnancy and Postpartum Hormonal Changes

Pregnancy triggers a flurry of hormone changes meant to feed and sustain the developing baby. To keep the pregnancy going, levels of human chorionic gonadotropin (hCG), progesterone, and estrogen increase. This biochemical alteration can affect not just appetite, but also how the body stores and utilizes energy.

Postpartum hormonal fluctuations continue as the body adapts to breastfeeding and healing. Breastfeeding, in particular, may increase calorie requirements. Maintaining a balanced diet to support both the mother's health and the infant's nutritional requirements is critical in managing these changes.

Managing Hormonal Shifts

Understanding the body's incredible adaptability is necessary for navigating hormonal fluctuations throughout the female experience. Regular physical activity, stress management, and mindful eating may all help to balance mood, energy, and metabolism during hormonal changes. To enhance their well-being at every stage of life, women must listen to their bodies, seek assistance when necessary, and make informed choices.

Menopause and Aging

Hormonal Changes and Wellness in Menopause and Aging

Women go through numerous phases of hormonal change during their lives, the most important of which is menopause. This natural shift, which is typically accompanied by the broader aging process, introduces significant physiological changes and ramifications. Understanding menopause and the aging process is essential for women's health and longevity.

The Menopause Milestone

Menopause usually occurs between the ages of 40 and 50 in women, however, this might vary. It is defined as the lack of menstruation for 12 months. This notable occurrence is distinguished by a reduction in the production of two important hormones: estrogen and progesterone. These hormonal changes have far-reaching implications:

Hot flashes and night sweats are frequent female symptoms that may disrupt sleep and daily life.

- ***Bone Health:*** A reduction in estrogen has been related to an increased risk of osteoporosis, a bone-weakening illness. Bone health may become a priority via diet, exercise, and supplementation.

- ***Mood Changes:*** Hormonal fluctuations during menopause may alter mood, causing symptoms such as impatience, anxiety, and sorrow. Alternative treatments or hormone replacement therapy (HRT) are options.

- ***Changes in metabolism and body*** composition may make gaining weight easier, especially around the abdomen. Regular exercise and a well-balanced diet constitute critical weight-management techniques.

- ***Cardiovascular Health:*** As estrogen levels decline, so does the risk of cardiovascular illness. Monitoring cardiovascular health via lifestyle choices and regular check-ups is crucial.

Aging gracefully

Other aging processes that affect both men and women are usually associated with menopause. These are some of the procedures:

- *Muscle Loss:* As we age, our muscle mass gradually reduces, which might lower our metabolism. Strength training and adequate protein ingestion are becoming more important.

- *Changes in Metabolic Rate:* The amount of calories burned at rest, known as basal metabolic rate (BMR), tends to decrease with age. This suggests that maintaining a healthy weight may include modifications in food and physical activity.

- *Hormonal Alterations:* Hormonal changes impact women even beyond menopause. Low amounts of growth hormone, for example, might affect muscle tone and energy levels.

- *Cognitive Health:* As we become older, we may notice cognitive changes such as minor memory lapses. Mental fitness routines and a brain-healthy diet may help improve cognitive well-being.

Chronic diseases, such as diabetes and certain cancers, grow increasingly frequent as individuals age. Prevention requires regular health checkups and appropriate lifestyle choices.

Coping with Menopause and Aging

Accepting natural processes while actively controlling their impact on health and well-being is required throughout menopause and aging. Here are some helpful hints for your journey:

- *Adopt a nutrient-dense,* well-balanced diet, engage in regular physical activity, decrease stress, and get adequate sleep.
- *Hormone Replacement Therapy (HRT):* To ease menopausal symptoms, some women choose hormone replacement therapy (HRT) under the guidance of a doctor. Consult a healthcare professional about the dangers and benefits.
- *Regular health check-ups aid* in the early detection and management of age-related health concerns.
- *Mental and emotional well-being:* Make mental health a priority by using stress-reduction techniques, maintaining social ties, and seeking professional assistance as needed.
- *Bone Health:* Get adequate calcium and vitamin D, and seek bone density testing and treatments if necessary.

Thyroid Function

The Master Regulator of Metabolism

The thyroid gland is a little, butterfly-shaped gland at the front of your neck that has a significant impact on your overall health. The thyroid is the key regulator of your metabolism, although it is often overlooked. Understanding thyroid function is critical for comprehending how this little gland can influence everything from energy levels to body weight and even mood.

The Thyroid's Role in Metabolism

The thyroid gland produces two essential hormones: thyroxine (T4) and triiodothyronine (T3). These hormones are critical in controlling the body's metabolic rate—the rate at which your cells convert food into energy. Here's how it works:

- ***Hormone Production:*** The thyroid gland is continually monitoring the body's energy needs. When your metabolism needs to be boosted, your thyroid generates more T4, an inactive form of thyroid hormone.

- ***Conversion to Active Form:*** The majority of T4 in the body is converted into T3, the active form of the hormone, in a variety of tissues, the most important of which is the liver.

- ***T3 travels via the bloodstream*** and into cells, where it binds to receptors on the cell's nucleus. This mechanism turns on genes involved in energy synthesis and metabolism.

- ***As T3 levels increase*** and energy needs are met, the thyroid gland receives signals to reduce T4 production, enabling a delicate balance to be maintained.

Common thyroid Disorders

Thyroid function may go wrong in several ways, causing health issues:

- *Hypothyroidism* occurs when the thyroid gland does not produce enough thyroid hormones. Common symptoms include fatigue, weight gain, melancholy, and a sense of being cold. The most common cause is Hashimoto's thyroiditis, an autoimmune disorder.

- *When the thyroid overproduces thyroid hormones*, it causes symptoms such as anxiety, rapid heartbeat, weight loss, and heat sensitivity. Graves disease is one of the most common causes of hyperthyroidism.

- *Thyroid Nodules:* Thyroid nodules are lumps or abnormal growths in the thyroid gland. While the majority are innocuous, a few are dangerous.

- *Thyroiditis:* Thyroid inflammation, which is usually caused by viral infections or autoimmune illnesses, may cause transient thyroid dysfunction as well as symptoms such as neck stiffness and fever.

Thyroid Disease Management

Thyroid health management comprises several key components:

Thyroid Function Testing: Regular thyroid function testing, which includes TSH (thyroid-stimulating hormone), T3, and T4 readings, may identify thyroid problems. The importance of early diagnosis and treatment cannot be overstated.

- **Medication:** Synthetic thyroid hormone replacement therapy (levothyroxine) is often used to treat hypothyroidism. Hyperthyroidism may be treated with medication, radioactive iodine treatment, or surgery.
- **Diet:** Thyroid function is dependent on nutrient-rich diets, notably those heavy in iodine, selenium, and zinc. Dietary restrictions, such as restricting goitrogenic foods that interfere with thyroid function, may be suggested in certain cases.
- **Chronic stress** may affect thyroid function. Yoga, meditation, and exercise may all be excellent stress-reduction techniques.
- **A healthy lifestyle** that includes regular exercise, enough sleep, and a well-balanced diet helps overall thyroid and metabolic health.

Lean Body Mass and Fat Storage

Balancing the Scales of Health

The relationship between lean body mass and fat growth is critical to overall health. While fat is required for energy storage and insulation, lean body mass (muscles, bones, and organs) is the body's metabolic powerhouse. Understanding this dynamic interaction is essential for maintaining a healthy and balanced body.

Lean Body Mass Is the Metabolic Engine

Everything in your body, except fat, is made up of lean body mass, also known as muscle mass. There are bones, organs, and, of course, muscles. Here's why it's so important:

Metabolism: Lean body mass is metabolically active tissue. It burns more calories than fat at rest. Individuals with a greater percentage of lean body mass have a higher basal metabolic rate (BMR), allowing them to burn more calories even when not exercising.

Muscle strength and mobility: Muscles provide the necessary strength and power for everyday activities. Maintaining lean body mass is crucial for maintaining mobility and functional independence.

Hormonal Balance: Hormones, particularly insulin sensitivity, are regulated by muscle tissue. Muscle mass may assist regulate blood sugar and reduce the risk of type 2 diabetes.

Fat Storage as a Source of Energy

Fat is another vital component of the body, however, it is mostly used for energy storage. Its purpose is as follows:

- *Excess calories* are stored in the form of triglycerides in the fat. When the body needs energy, it may use these fat stores.

- ***Insulation and protection:*** Fat works as insulation, contributing to body temperature control. It also serves as a cushion and shields vital organs.
- ***Hormone Production:*** Hormones like leptin and adiponectin are generated by fat tissue and help with appetite control and insulin sensitivity.

The Lean Body Mass to Fat Mass Ratio

Achieving optimal health often entails establishing a balance between lean body mass and fat accumulation. Excess body fat, especially around the abdomen, has been related to an increased risk of metabolic diseases such as heart disease and diabetes. Extremely low body fat, on the other hand, may lead to health issues including hormone imbalances and lowered immunity.

Methods for Keeping Lean Body Mass While Reducing Fat Storage

Strength Training: Regular resistance or strength training exercises are required for the development and maintenance of lean body mass. These exercises include weight lifting, bodyweight training, and resistance bands.

Cardiovascular activity, such as running, swimming, or cycling, aids in calorie burn and fat loss.

Consume a diet rich in lean meats, whole grains, fruits, and vegetables. Protein intake is particularly important for maintaining and developing lean body mass.

Caloric Balance: To maintain or lose weight, calorie intake and expenditure must be balanced. You may achieve this balance by keeping track of your calorie intake and expenditure.

Adequate Rest and Sleep: Adequate rest and sleep are critical for muscle recovery and overall health.

Chronic stress may lead to fat accumulation, especially around the abdomen. Stress-reduction techniques such as mindfulness, yoga, and meditation may help.

Regular health check-ups may assist you in assessing your body composition, metabolism, and overall wellness.

Emotional and psychological factors

The Mind-Body Connection and Health

The significance of emotional and psychological factors in physical health cannot be overstated. Our thoughts, emotions, and mental health all have an impact on our physical health, and vice versa. Understanding this intricate link is essential for achieving overall well-being.

The Mind-Body Connection

The mind-body link refers to the delicate relationship between mental and emotional states and physical health. It focuses on how our thoughts, emotions, and actions may affect our physical health and vice versa. Here's how it works:

- When you are stressed, your body reacts with a "fight or flight" reaction, which might be caused by a demanding job, relationship problems, or other circumstances. This leads the body to produce stress chemicals like cortisol and adrenaline, which may have several effects on the body, ranging from raising blood pressure to hindering digestion.

- Chronic stress may weaken your immune system, making you more susceptible to illnesses and infections. Positive emotions and a strong feeling of well-being, on the other hand, may boost your immune system's effectiveness.

- Emotional and psychological factors may influence how you perceive and manage pain. Chronic pain, in particular, is usually linked to mental distress.

- Emotional states can influence behavior, such as food habits, physical activity, and sleep patterns. Stress, for example, may result in emotional eating or a lack of sleep, negatively influencing overall health.

Factors Influencing Emotional and Psychological Health

Several emotional and psychological difficulties may have an impact on physical health:

- Chronic stress has been related to several health problems, including cardiovascular disease, digestive issues, and mental health issues.

- Anxiety and depression may affect energy levels, sleep, appetite, and the immune system.

- Chronic Emotional States: Persistent negative emotions, such as fury or resentment, may lead to physical health issues over time.

- Body Image and Self-Esteem: Your opinion of yourself and your body may impact your lifestyle choices, such as diet, exercise, and self-care.

Methods for Strengthening the Mind-Body Bond

- Stress Management: Practice stress reduction practices such as meditation, deep breathing exercises, yoga, or mindfulness to minimize the effect of chronic stress on physical health.

- Endorphins, which are natural mood lifters, are released after physical exertion. It may also help with stress reduction and sleeping better.

- Healthy Eating Habits: Nutrition is critical for both mental and physical health. A well-balanced, nutrient-dense diet improves both mental and physical well-being.

- Sleep hygiene is crucial since it aids in emotional control and overall well-being.

- Maintain close social connections with friends and family to provide emotional support and to relieve feelings of isolation or loneliness.

- Therapy and counseling: Seek professional help when needed, particularly if you are coping with conditions like depression, anxiety, or chronic stress.

- Mindfulness Practices: Increase self-awareness and emotional balance by engaging in mindfulness-promoting activities such as meditation or journaling.

- Develop healthy relationships that provide emotional support and promote well-being.

- Make self-care activities that promote relaxation and emotional balance a priority, such as reading, hobbies, or time spent outdoors.

METABOLIC CONFUSION APPROACH

What is Metabolic Confusion?

Metabolic Confusion is a dietary and lifestyle approach that improves metabolism and promotes weight control by causing purposeful changes in calorie intake, macronutrient composition, and meal timing. This strategy aims to prevent the body from reacting to a set schedule, which may result in weight plateaus and lower metabolic efficiency.

Here's an in-depth study of Metabolic Confusion:

- **Strategic Caloric Variations:** To treat metabolic confusion, calorie intake should be cycled, with periods of higher and lower calorie consumption. This adjustment is intended to prevent the body from reacting to a constant calorie level, which might impair metabolism.

- **Macronutrient Manipulation:** One typical method is to change the balance of macronutrients in your diet, such as the carbohydrate, protein, and fat ratios. This difference may affect how the body processes and uses certain nutrients.

- **Metabolic Confusion may be treated with intermittent fasting** or by changing meal times. For example, you may alternate between days with longer fasting periods and days with regular eating patterns. This mutation has the potential to impact insulin sensitivity and fat metabolism.

- **Physical Activity Integration:** Physical activity is a key component of Metabolic Confusion. Strength training, cardiovascular exercise, and high-intensity interval training (HIIT) are all common elements. Changing your training program prevents your body from adjusting to a certain exercise pattern.

- **Hormonal Considerations:** Metabolic Confusion takes into account the influence of hormones on metabolism, including insulin and cortisol. Dietary and stress management measures are often employed to control these hormones.

- **Periodization:** The strategy is typically organized in cycles, with you following one plan for a specific period (e.g., a few weeks) before moving to another. This cycle may help the body stay flexible to change.

Women benefit from metabolic confusion.

Women may benefit from Metabolic Confusion since it targets their specific physiological and hormonal concerns. Here are some specific ways this method might help women:

- Hormonal Balance: Variations in women's hormones, particularly throughout the menstrual cycle, may influence appetite, energy levels, and metabolism. Metabolic Confusion may help you synchronize your food and exercise programs with these hormonal swings, resulting in better hormonal balance throughout the month.

- Metabolic Confusion may help women break through weight loss plateaus and increase fat loss by consciously changing calorie intake, macronutrient ratios, and meal timing. This strategy stops the body from responding to a certain eating plan, resulting in efficient fat-burning.

- Long-Term Weight Management: Unlike strict, short-term diets, Metabolic Confusion emphasizes lifestyle adjustments. In the long run, this makes it more sustainable for women, reducing the possibility of yo-yo dieting and weight regain.

- Increased Insulin Sensitivity: Some Metabolic Confusion variations concentrate on insulin regulation, which may be particularly beneficial for women who are insulin-resistant or at risk of developing type 2 diabetes.

- Menopause Support: As women age and reach menopause, their metabolism alters. Metabolic Confusion may help address these metabolic changes, promoting weight management and overall health during this stage of life.

- Muscle Preservation: The strategy typically incorporates strength training and resistance exercises, which are essential for keeping lean body mass. Women may reverse age-related muscle loss, particularly via strength training.

- Individualization: Metabolic Confusion may be adjusted to match the needs and preferences of each person. Women may tailor their approach to their metabolic demands, resulting in a more customized and adaptive strategy.

- Psychological Benefits: Metabolic Confusion's adaptive approach helps ease the strain and concern that might be associated with strict diets. This can enhance women's mental and emotional health by fostering a positive connection with food and body image.

- Encourages a Diverse Diet: Women may have unique nutritional requirements, particularly during pregnancy and nursing. Metabolic Confusion encourages a diversified diet, which may help women achieve their nutritional needs more effectively.

Metabolic Perplexity: A Scientific Look

Metabolic Confusion is founded on knowledge of metabolism, physiology, and nutrition. This strategy tries to increase metabolism and promote weight reduction by continually challenging the body with variations in calorie intake, macronutrient composition, and meal timing. The scientific concepts supporting Metabolic Confusion are as follows:

- Adaptive Thermogenesis: The human body is very adaptable. When you eat a certain number of calories consistently and stick to the same diet and exercise habits, your body tends to adapt to that pattern. Your metabolism may decrease with time, making it more difficult to lose or maintain weight. Metabolic Confusion disrupts this adaptation by periodically changing calorie intake and macronutrient ratios, preventing the body from being caught in a metabolic rut.

- Hormonal Influence: Hormones have a vital role in metabolism and fat formation. Metabolic Confusion takes into account the effects of hormones such as insulin, cortisol, and leptin. Intermittent fasting, which is used in numerous Metabolic Confusion approaches, may improve insulin sensitivity, which is required for successful fat-burning and blood sugar control.

- Thermic Effect of Dietary (TEF): TEF refers to the quantity of energy consumed by the body to digest, absorb, and metabolize dietary components. The TEF values for different macronutrients vary. Protein, for example, has a higher TEF than carbohydrates or lipids, indicating that it requires more energy to digest. Variations in macronutrient intake are widely utilized to modulate the TEF and perhaps boost calorie expenditure in Metabolic Confusion.

- Muscle Preservation: Muscle, especially, is a metabolically active tissue. Muscle maintenance and development are vital for maintaining a healthy metabolism. Strength training, which is an important part of many Metabolic Confusion programs, helps to maintain and develop muscle mass, which may lead to greater resting calorie expenditure.

- Psychological and Behavioral Factors: Metabolic Confusion emphasizes the role of psychology in diet compliance and success. Changing meal plans and exercise routines regularly may assist in reducing the monotony and boredom associated with restrictive diets, making them more psychologically sustainable.

- Periodization: Metabolic Confusion typically uses periodization, a sports training method. It comprises switching between different foods and workout regimens to challenge the body in new ways. Periodization may help optimize metabolic adaptability while reducing the chance of plateaus.

- While research in this area is continuing, some studies suggest that intermittent fasting and calorie adjustments may have metabolic and health benefits, such as improved insulin sensitivity and fat loss. Individual responses, however, may vary.

DEVELOPING YOUR METABOLIC CONFUSION PLAN

Setting up a Metabolic Confusion Diet

A Metabolic Confusion diet comprises making deliberate alterations to calorie intake, macronutrient composition, and meal timing. This strategy aims to boost metabolism and ease weight reduction. Here is a step-by-step guide to designing a Metabolic Confusion diet.

Establish Specific Objectives:

- Define your particular goals, whether they be weight reduction, muscle growth, or improved metabolic health.
- Take into consideration your dietary preferences, limitations, and any underlying medical conditions.

Determine Your Caloric Requirements

- Calculate your daily calorie needs based on age, gender, activity level, and goals. For more accuracy, use online calculators or see a registered dietitian.
- Break down your calorie goal into daily or weekly objectives. For example, if your daily calorie target is 2,000, you may aim for 1,800 calories on certain days and 2,200 calories on others.

Macronutrient Variations:

- Create a plan for changing macronutrient ratios. For example, on certain days, you may eat more calories from carbohydrates while concentrating on protein or healthy fats.
- Check your protein intake to ensure that you are getting enough to support muscle maintenance and metabolism.

Meal Scheduling

- Include intermittent fasting or mealtime modifications in your plan. For example, you may alternate between days with a 16/8 fasting schedule (16 hours of fasting and 8 hours of eating) and days with typical meal patterns.
- Experiment with when you have your biggest meal. Some types of Metabolic Confusion suggest eating your biggest meal first thing in the morning.

Calorie Intake During a Cycle

- Calorie cycling should be practiced throughout the week. For example:
- High-calorie days: Increase your calorie intake to achieve a surplus. This may promote muscle growth and metabolism.
- Low-calorie days: Consume fewer calories to create a calorie deficit, which encourages fat loss.

- Maintenance calories: On maintenance days, consume maintenance calories to allow your body to relax from calorie fluctuations.

Components of exercise:

- Include a variety of fitness types in your everyday program. Strength training, aerobics, and high-intensity interval training (HIIT) are all advised.
- To keep your body guessing, vary the intensity, duration, and kind of exercise.

Track your progress:

- Keep note of your food and exercise habits, as well as your progress towards your objectives.
- Keep note of how your body responds to different calorie and macronutrient changes. Adapt your plan depending on the results.

Stay hydrated:

- Hydration is essential for metabolic and overall health. Make sure you drink enough water throughout the day.

Sufficient Nutrition:

- To meet your nutritional needs, consider nutrient-dense foods. Eat a variety of fruits and vegetables, as well as lean proteins, whole grains, and healthy fats.

Remain Consistent and Patient:

- Metabolic confusion cannot be resolved quickly. Long-term success depends on consistency and patience. Maintain your focus on your objective and do not be discouraged by short-term fluctuations.

Effective Meal Plans for Women

Day 1: High-Calory Day (Maintenance)

Breakfast:

- Scrambled eggs with spinach and tomatoes.
- Whole-grain toast
- Greek yogurt with berries.

Lunch:

- Grilled chicken salad with mixed greens, cucumbers, bell peppers, and a vinaigrette dressing.

Snack:

- A handful of mixed nuts

Dinner:

- baked salmon with quinoa
- Steamed broccoli.

Day 2: Low Calorie Day (Deficit)

Breakfast:

- Smoothie with spinach, banana, almond milk, and protein powder

Lunch

- Lentil soup with a side salad.

Snack:

- Carrot sticks and hummus.

Dinner:

A grilled turkey burger covered in lettuce leaves.

- Roasted sweet potatoes

Day 3: Moderate Calorie Day (Maintenance)

Breakfast:

- Overnight oatmeal with almond milk, chia seeds, and mixed berries.

Lunch:

- Tuna salad served with mixed greens, cherry tomatoes, olives, and a mild dressing.

Snack:

- Apple slices with peanut butter.

Dinner:

- Stir-fried tofu with mixed veggies and brown rice.

Day 4: Low Calorie Day (Deficit)

Breakfast:

- Greek yogurt parfait made with oats and mixed fruit

Lunch:

- Mixed greens salad with grilled shrimp and a mild vinaigrette dressing.

Snack:

- Cucumber slices with hummus.

Dinner:

- Baked chicken breast with roasted broccoli.

Day 5: Moderate Calorie Day (Maintenance)

Breakfast:

- Vegetable and cheese omelet
- Whole-grain toast

Lunch:

- Quinoa salad made with black beans, corn, and a lime-cilantro dressing

Snack:

- Sliced mango sprinkled with chile powder

Dinner:

- Grilled steak with sautéed spinach and quinoa.

Day 6 - High Calorie Day (Maintenance)

Breakfast:

- Scrambled eggs with diced tomatoes and avocado.
- Whole-grain toast

Lunch:

- Chickpea and vegetable curry with brown rice.

Snack:

- A mixture of nuts and dry fruit

Dinner:

- Baked cod in lemon butter sauce
- Roasted asparagus.

Day 7: Low Calorie Day (Deficit)

Breakfast:

- Protein smoothie made with spinach, banana, almond milk, and a scoop of protein powder.

Lunch:

- Mixed green salad with grilled chicken breast and a mild vinaigrette dressing

Snack:

- Bell pepper slices with tzatziki dip.

Dinner:

- Baked salmon with lemon and herbs
- Steamed broccoli.

Week 2:

Day 8 - High Calorie Day (Maintenance)

Breakfast:

- Omelet made with mushrooms, spinach, and feta cheese
- Whole-grain toast
- Sliced avocado.

Lunch:

- Quinoa salad with chickpeas, sliced cucumber, cherry tomatoes, and a lemon-tahini vinaigrette.

Snack:

- Mixed berries and cottage cheese

Dinner:

- Grilled shrimp skewers and brown rice
- Steamed asparagus.

Day 9: Low Calorie Day (Deficit)

Breakfast:

- Greek yogurt with honey and chopped almonds.

Lunch:

- Mixed bean salad with red onions, bell peppers, and a mild balsamic vinaigrette.

Snack:

- Celery sticks with hummus.

Dinner:

- Baked chicken breast with roasted Brussels sprouts.

Day 10: Moderate Calorie Day (Maintenance)

Breakfast:

- Protein smoothie made with spinach, banana, almond milk, and chia seeds.

Lunch:

- Chicken breasts filled with spinach and feta
- Quinoa and sautéed kale

Snack:

- Pear slices with ricotta cheese.

Dinner:

- baked cod with lemon and herbs
- Steamed broccoli.

Day 11 - High Calorie Day (Maintenance)

Breakfast:

- Scrambled eggs with chopped bell peppers, onions
- Whole-grain toast
- Mixed-berry compote

Lunch:

- Bowl of grilled vegetables and quinoa with tahini dressing

Snack:

- Sliced apples with almond butter.

Dinner:

- Beef stir-fry with carrots, broccoli, and brown rice

Day 12: Low Calorie Day (Deficit)

Breakfast:

- Cottage cheese and pineapple chunks.

Lunch:

- Spinach and mixed greens salad with grilled chicken breast and balsamic vinaigrette.

Snack:

- Cherry tomatoes with mozzarella cheese.

Dinner:

- Baked salmon with lemon and dill.
- Steamed green beans

Day 13: Moderate Calorie Day (Maintenance)

Breakfast:

- Overnight oatmeal with almond milk, sliced bananas, and chopped walnuts

Lunch:

- Tofu and vegetable stir fry with quinoa

Snack:

- Mixed nuts and dried fruit

Dinner:

- Grilled turkey meatballs with whole-grain spaghetti and marinara sauce.

Day 14 - High Calorie Day (Maintenance)

Breakfast:

- Protein pancakes topped with fresh berries and a scoop of Greek yogurt

Lunch:

- Lentil and vegetable soup served with a side salad

Snack:

- Baby carrots with tzatziki dip.

Dinner:

- Baked chicken thighs with roasted sweet potatoes and Brussels sprouts.

Week 3:

Day 15 - High Calorie Day (Maintenance)

Breakfast:

- Scrambled eggs with spinach and chopped tomatoes
- Whole-grain toast
- Greek yogurt with honey.

Lunch:

- Grilled chicken and quinoa dish, mixed veggies, and a light vinaigrette dressing

Snack:

- Mixed berries with cottage cheese

Dinner:

- Baked salmon with quinoa
- Steamed asparagus.

Day 16: Low Calorie Day (Deficit)

Breakfast:

- Protein smoothie includes kale, banana, almond milk, and a scoop of protein powder.

Lunch:

- Lentil soup with a side salad.

Snack:

- Cucumber slices with hummus

Dinner:

- A grilled turkey burger covered in lettuce leaves.
- roasted sweet potatoes

Day 17: Moderate-Calore Day (Maintenance)

Breakfast:

- Overnight oatmeal with almond milk, chia seeds, and mixed berries.

Lunch:

- Tuna salad served with mixed greens, cherry tomatoes, olives, and a mild dressing.

Snack:

- Apple slices with almond butter.

Dinner:

- Stir-fried tofu with mixed veggies and brown rice.

Day 18 - High Calorie Day (Maintenance)

Breakfast:

- Omelette made with mushrooms, bell peppers, and feta cheese
- Whole-grain toast
- Sliced avocado.

Lunch:

- Quinoa salad with chickpeas, sliced cucumber, cherry tomatoes, and a lemon-tahini vinaigrette.

Snack:

- Handful of assorted nuts.

Dinner:

- Beef stir-fry with carrots, broccoli, and brown rice

Day 19: Low Calorie Day (Deficit)

Breakfast:

- Greek yogurt with honey and chopped almonds.

Lunch:

- Mixed bean salad with red onions, bell peppers, and a mild balsamic vinaigrette.

Snack:

- Carrot sticks with hummus

Dinner:

- Baked chicken breast with roasted Brussels sprouts.

Day 20: Moderate-Calore Day (Maintenance)

Breakfast:

- Protein smoothie made with spinach, banana, almond milk, and chia seeds.

Lunch:

- Chicken breast stuffed with spinach and feta.
- Quinoa and sautéed kale

Snack:

- Mixed nuts and dried fruit

Dinner:

- Grilled turkey meatballs with whole-grain spaghetti and marinara sauce.

Day 21: High-Calory Day (Maintenance)

Breakfast:

- Scrambled eggs with chopped bell peppers, onions

- Whole-grain toast
- Mixed-berry compote

Lunch:

- Lentil and vegetable soup served with a side salad

Snack:

- Sliced apples with peanut butter.

Dinner:

- Baked chicken thighs with roasted sweet potatoes and Brussels sprouts.

Day 22

Breakfast:

- Greek yogurt parfait made with oats and mixed fruit

Lunch:

- Mixed greens salad with grilled shrimp and a mild vinaigrette dressing.

Snack:

- Cucumber slices with hummus.

Dinner:

- Baked chicken breast with roasted broccoli.

Day 23

Breakfast:

- Scrambled eggs with diced tomatoes and avocado.
- Whole-grain toast

Lunch:

- Chickpea and vegetable curry with brown rice.

Snack:

- A mixture of nuts and dry fruit

Dinner:

- Baked cod in lemon butter sauce
- Roasted asparagus.

Day 24

Breakfast:

- Greek yogurt with honey and chopped almonds.

Lunch:

- Mixed bean salad with red onions, bell peppers, and a mild balsamic vinaigrette.

Snack:

- Celery sticks with hummus.

Dinner:

- Baked chicken breast with roasted Brussels sprouts.

Day 25

Breakfast:

- Scrambled eggs with chopped bell peppers, onions
- Whole-grain toast
- Mixed-berry compote

Lunch:

- Bowl of grilled vegetables and quinoa with tahini dressing

Snack:

- Sliced apples with almond butter.

Dinner:

- Beef stir-fry with carrots, broccoli, and brown rice

Day 26

Breakfast:

- Overnight oatmeal with almond milk, sliced bananas, and chopped walnuts

Lunch:

- Tofu and vegetable stir fry with quinoa

Snack:

- Mixed nuts and dried fruit

Dinner:

- Grilled turkey meatballs with whole-grain spaghetti and marinara sauce.

Day 27

Breakfast:

- Scrambled eggs with spinach and chopped tomatoes
- Whole-grain toast
- Greek yogurt with honey.

Lunch:

- Grilled chicken and quinoa dish, mixed veggies, and a light vinaigrette dressing

Snack:

- Mixed berries with cottage cheese

Dinner:

- Baked salmon with quinoa
- Steamed asparagus.

Day 28:

Breakfast:

- Overnight oatmeal with almond milk, chia seeds, and mixed berries.

Lunch:

- Tuna salad served with mixed greens, cherry tomatoes, olives, and a mild dressing.

Snack:

- Apple slices with almond butter.

Dinner:

- Stir-fried tofu with mixed veggies and brown rice.

Day 29

Breakfast:

- Greek yogurt with honey and chopped almonds.

Lunch:

- Mixed bean salad with red onions, bell peppers, and a mild balsamic vinaigrette.

Snack:

- Carrot sticks with hummus

Dinner:

- Baked chicken breast with roasted Brussels sprouts.

Day 30

Breakfast:

- Scrambled eggs with chopped bell peppers, onions
- Whole-grain toast
- Mixed-berry compote

Lunch:

- Lentil and vegetable soup served with a side salad

Snack:

- Sliced apples with peanut butter.

Dinner:

- Baked chicken thighs with roasted sweet potatoes and Brussels sprouts.

Integrating Metabolic Confusion Strategies

Incorporating Metabolic Confusion Strategies into Your Lifestyle entails taking a deliberate and multifaceted approach to optimizing your metabolism and supporting your health and fitness goals. Here's a more comprehensive guide for effectively integrating these strategies:

- *Caloric Variation:* Change your daily calorie intake regularly. Incorporate days with higher calorie consumption that are roughly equal to your maintenance level. Alternate between days with a calorie deficit for weight management and days with your normal intake.

- *Macronutrient Manipulation:* Change your macronutrient ratios. On certain days, focus on carbohydrates, while on others, increase your protein or healthy fat intake. For balanced nutrition, ensure that you consume a diverse range of macronutrients.

- *Meal Timing:* Experiment with different meal timing patterns, such as intermittent fasting or structured eating windows. For example, on some days, limit your eating time to 8 hours and allow for a 16-hour fast.

- *Incorporate variety into your exercise routine.* Incorporate strength training, cardiovascular workouts, and high-intensity interval training (HIIT). To keep your body challenged, switch up the intensity, duration, and types of exercises you do.

- *Hormone Management:* Pay close attention to hormonal fluctuations, particularly those affecting metabolism. Incorporate dietary strategies that promote hormonal balance, such as choosing foods that regulate insulin and cortisol levels.

- *Periodization:* Include cycling in your plan. Follow a specific diet and exercise plan for several weeks before switching to a different one. This approach keeps your body from adapting to a set routine.

- *Monitor and Adjust:* Keep a detailed journal of your progress, including your eating habits and exercise routines. Analyze how your body reacts to various strategies, and be prepared to make changes based on your findings.

- *Stay Hydrated:* Proper hydration is essential to a healthy metabolism. Drink plenty of water throughout the day to maintain overall health and metabolic processes.

- *To meet your body's nutritional* needs, prioritize nutrient-dense foods such as fresh fruits and vegetables, lean proteins, whole grains, and healthy fats.

- *Adequate Sleep:* Recognize the significance of good sleep. Sufficient and restful sleep is essential for hormonal balance and a healthy metabolism.

- *Mindful Eating:* Develop mindful eating practices. Listen to your body's hunger and fullness cues, and avoid impulsive or emotionally driven eating habits.

- *Consistency is Essential:* Keep in mind that Metabolic Confusion is not a quick fix. Long-term success depends on unwavering consistency. Stick to your plan, be patient, and keep in mind that long-term results often require time.

A COLLECTION OF RECIPES FOR WOMEN'S HEALTHY METABOLIC CONFUSION

Sweet Potato with Spinach and Mushroom Stuffing

Ingredients:

- Two huge sweet potatoes.
- Fresh spinach, two cups.
- 1 cup of sliced mushrooms.
- 1/4 cup crumbled feta cheese.
- Olive oil, 1 tablespoon, pepper, and salt to taste

Instructions:

- Heat the oven to 400 degrees Fahrenheit (200 degrees Celsius).
- You should clean the sweet potatoes, then fork them, and then bake them for forty-five to sixty minutes, or until they are tender.
- In a saucepan, olive oil is brought up to a temperature that is somewhere in the middle. Sauté the mushrooms until they become brown and release moisture, then add them to the pan and continue to cook them.
- The spinach should be cooked in the pan until it has become wilted.

- After cutting each sweet potato in half, fluff the flesh of each sweet potato with a fork, and then place the mushroom-spinach combination on top of the sweet potato.

- After seasoning with salt and pepper, sprinkle feta cheese over top.

Nutrient Info (per Serving):

- 265 calories

- 8g protein

- 45g of carbohydrates

- 9g of dietary fiber

- 6g sugars

- Fat: 9g

- 352% vitamin A DV

- 35% vitamin C DV

Salad with quinoa and black beans

Ingredients:

- One cup of cooked quinoa

- One can (15 oz) Drain and wash black beans

- 1 cup of cherry tomatoes, cut in half

- Frozen or fresh corn kernels, half a cup

- 1/4 cup red onion, diced coarsely

- 1/4 cup of freshly chopped cilantro

- The juice of one lime

- Two tsp each of pepper and salt, plus olive oil, to taste

Instructions:

- In a large bowl, mix cooked quinoa, black beans, cherry tomatoes, corn, red onion, and cilantro.
- In a separate small dish, mix lime juice, olive oil, salt, and pepper to make the dressing.
- Drizzle the dressing over the salad and toss to combine.

Nutrient Info (per Serving):

- 284 calories
- 8g protein
- 46g of carbohydrates
- 8g of dietary fiber
- 5g sugars
- Fat: 8g
- 40% of vitamin C. Iron: 15% DV DV

A parfait of Greek yogurt

Ingredients:

- One cup of Greek yogurt, low or no-fat
- 1/2 cup of raspberries, blueberries, and strawberries combined
- One teaspoon each of honey or maple syrup
- Double-spooned granola.

Instructions:

- In a glass or plate, combine Greek yogurt, mixed berries, honey or maple syrup, and granola.
- Repetition of the layers is possible.
- Present cold.

Nutrient Info (per Serving):

- 252 calories
- 15g of protein
- 37g of carbohydrates
- 6g of dietary fiber
- 26g sugars
- Fat: 6g
- DV calcium: 22%
- 22% DV of vitamin C

Stir-fried vegetables and chickpeas

Ingredients:

- One cup of cooked chickpeas
- Two cups of mixed vegetables, such as broccoli, bell peppers, snap peas, and carrots
- one finely chopped clove of garlic
- One tablespoon of sesame oil, one teaspoon of low-sodium soy sauce

- 1/8 tsp finely chopped ginger

- Red pepper flakes (optional)

- Brown rice or cooked quinoa, as preferred (for serving).

Instructions:

- In a large pan, the sesame oil should be heated to medium heat. Add the ginger and garlic and sauté for 1 minute.

- Add the mixed vegetables and stir-fry until they become crisp-tender.

- Add the chickpeas and soy sauce, and cook for a further two to three minutes.

- Serve the recipe over brown rice or cooked quinoa, if you'd like.

Nutritional Info (per serving, not including rice or quinoa):

- 222 calories

- 8g of protein

- 23g of carbohydrates

- 7g of dietary fiber

- 6g of sugar,

- 10g of fat

- 17% DV for iron

- 85% DV of vitamin C

Balsamic-vinaigrette-topped salad with berries and spinach

Ingredients:

- Fresh spinach greens, two cups
- Strawberries, blueberries, and raspberries equal 1/2 cup.
- 1/4 cup crumbled Feta cheese
- 1/4 cup of chopped walnuts.
- Balsamic vinegar, 2 tablespoons
- Combine olive oil, 1 tbsp honey, pepper, and salt to taste.

Instructions:

- A meal with walnuts, feta cheese, mixed berries, and fresh spinach is served.
- In a separate small dish, mix balsamic vinegar, olive oil, honey, salt, and pepper to make the dressing.
- Drizzle the dressing over the salad and toss again.

Nutrient Info (per Serving):

- 285 calories
- 7g of protein and 20g of carbohydrates
- 5g of dietary fiber
- 13g sugars
- Fat: 22g
- 75% DV for vitamin A
- 45% DV of vitamin C

Avocado and Black Bean Salad

Ingredients:

- one diced ripe avocado
- One can (15 oz) of rinsed and drained black beans
- One cup of kernel corn (fresh or frozen)
- 1/4 cup chopped red bell pepper
- two tablespoons freshly chopped cilantro and one lime's juice
- One tablespoon of olive oil
- To taste, add salt and pepper.

Instructions:

- Diced avocado, black beans, corn, red bell pepper, and cilantro should all be combined in a big dish.
- To make the dressing, combine the lime juice, olive oil, salt, and pepper in a small bowl.
- Over the salad, drizzle with the dressing and toss lightly to mix.

Nutritional Info (per serving):

- Calories: 285
- Protein: 8g
- Carbohydrates: 34g
- Dietary Fiber: 11g
- Sugars: 4g

- Fat: 13g

- Vitamin C: 46% DV

- Iron: 22% DV

Mediterranean Quinoa Bowl

Ingredients:

- One cup of cooked quinoa

- Half a cup of rinsed and drained chickpeas

- half a cup of chopped cucumbers

- Half a cup of cherry tomatoes

- 1/4 cup finely sliced red onion

- Two teaspoons of pitted and sliced Kalamata olives

- Two teaspoons of crumbled feta cheese

- One tablespoon of olive oil

- One-third cup of balsamic vinegar

- To taste, add salt and pepper.

Instructions:

- The quinoa that has been cooked, chickpeas, cucumber, cherry tomatoes, red onion, olives, and feta cheese should all be mixed in a bowl.

- The dressing is made by combining olive oil, balsamic vinegar, salt, and pepper in a small basin along with whisking them together.

- Coat the quinoa with the dressing by drizzling it over the bowl and then tossing it.

Nutritional Info (per serving):

- Calories: 322
- Protein: 10g
- Carbohydrates: 42g
- Dietary Fiber: 9g
- Sugars: 5g
- Fat: 11g
- Calcium: 16% DV
- Iron: 16% DV

Egg and Vegetable Stir-Fry

Ingredients:

- Two big eggs, beaten
- 1 cup mixed veggies (bell peppers, broccoli, carrots)
- 1 clove garlic, minced
- 1 tablespoon low-sodium soy sauce.
- 1/2 tablespoon of sesame oil.
- Cooked brown rice (optional, for serving)

Instructions:

- The sesame oil should be heated over medium-high heat in a pan that does not stick. Sauté the garlic for one minute after adding it.
- After adding the veggies, stir-fry them until they are soft.
- After pushing the veggies to one side of the pan, add the eggs that have been beaten to the other side of the skillet. Eggs should be scrambled.
- When the eggs have finished cooking, mix them with the veggies and then toss in the soy sauce into the mixture.
- If preferred, serve on brown rice that has been cooked.

Nutritional Info (per serving, excluding rice):

- Calories: 195
- Protein: 12g
- Carbohydrates: 8g
- Dietary Fiber: 3g
- Sugars: 4g
- Fat: 11g
- Iron: 11% DV
- Vitamin C: 45% DV

Berry Protein Smoothie Bowl

Ingredients:

- 1 cup of unsweetened almond milk.

- 1 scoop of vanilla protein powder.

- 1 cup mixed berries (strawberries, blueberries, raspberries)

- 1 ripe banana, cut, and 2 tablespoons chia seeds

- 1 tablespoon honey or maple syrup (optional)

- Toppings: sliced almonds, shredded coconut, fresh strawberries.

Instructions:

- The ingredients for this smoothie are as follows: almond milk, protein powder, mixed berries, banana, chia seeds, and honey or maple syrup if preferred. Blend until smooth. Blend until it is completely smooth.

- A bowl should be used to pour the smoothie, and then fresh berries, sliced almonds, and shredded coconut should be sprinkled on top.

Nutritional Info (per serving):

- Calories: 352

- Protein: 23g

- Carbohydrates: 46g

- Dietary Fiber: 13g

- Sugars: 24g

- Fat: 11g
- Calcium: 22% DV
- Vitamin C: 43% DV

Asian-Inspired Tofu and Vegetable Stir-Fry

Ingredients:

- One cubed block of extra-firm tofu
- Two cups of mixed veggies (broccoli, bell peppers, snap peas, carrots)
- two minced garlic cloves
- One-third cup of low-sodium soy sauce
- One tsp of hoisin sauce
- Half a tablespoon of sesame oil
- cooked quinoa or brown rice (optional, for serving)

Instructions:

- Cut the tofu into cubes after pressing it to remove extra water.
- Sesame oil should be heated over medium-high heat in a big skillet. Garlic is added and cooked for one minute.
- Stir-fry the tofu until it becomes golden brown.
- When the mixed veggies are tender, add them and stir-fry some more.
- Add hoisin sauce and soy sauce and stir.
- If preferred, serve over cooked quinoa or brown rice.

Nutritional Info (per serving, excluding rice/quinoa):

- Calories: 250
- Protein: 17g
- Carbohydrates: 25g
- Dietary Fiber: 7g
- Sugars: 7g
- Fat: 16g
- Iron: 25% DV
- Vitamin C: 85% DV

WOMEN EXERCISE

Function of Exercise

Exercise serves a variety of purposes in a woman's life and is essential for overall health, well-being, and quality of life. Exercise has several physical, mental, and emotional benefits that may enhance many aspects of a woman's life. The following is a thorough overview of the function of exercise.

1. Physical Fitness:

- Weight Control: Regular exercise helps you maintain a healthy weight by burning calories and increasing metabolism. When combined with a balanced diet, it may assist you in losing weight.

- Aerobic exercise, such as running, swimming, and cycling, improves cardiovascular fitness, lowers blood pressure, and reduces the risk of heart disease and stroke.

- Weight-bearing exercises and resistance training increase muscle hypertrophy, strength, and endurance. This may boost physical performance while decreasing the likelihood of injury.

- Weight-bearing exercises, such as walking or weightlifting, help to grow and maintain bone density, reducing the risk of osteoporosis and fractures.

- Joint Health: Exercises that include frequent, controlled movement, such as yoga and Pilates, may increase joint flexibility and reduce the risk of joint-related disorders such as arthritis.

- Immune System: Moderate exercise may help the body fight infections and disorders by strengthening its immune system.

2. Mental Wellbeing:

- Exercise triggers the release of endorphins, which are natural mood enhancers. It reduces stress, anxiety, and depression while enhancing overall mental health.

- Improved Sleep: Regular exercise may improve sleep quality and duration, leading to greater mental alertness and cognitive function.

- It has been proved that exercise improves memory, cognitive function, and attention. It has the potential to reduce the risk of cognitive decline and age-related conditions like dementia.

3. Emotional health:

- Confidence: Meeting workout goals and feeling physically strong may boost self-esteem and confidence.

- Social contact: Group fitness classes or team sports promote social interaction and the building of strong social bonds, reducing feelings of isolation.

4. Women's Specific Advantages:

- Regular exercise may help to alleviate monthly pain, reduce PMS symptoms, and improve overall menstrual health.

- Pregnancy and Postpartum: When done properly and under supervision, exercise throughout pregnancy may help with labor and recovery. Exercise after delivery may help you regain strength and vigor.

- Menopause: Exercise may help alleviate menopause symptoms including hot flashes, mood swings, and insomnia. It also helps bone health at this stage of life.

5. Lifespan:

- Lifespan Extension: Regular physical activity has been linked to living a longer and healthier life, lessening the risk of chronic diseases associated with aging.

6. Disease control:

- Exercise may help lower the risk of some types of cancer, including breast and colon cancer.

- Diabetes: Regular physical exercise may help diabetics avoid type 2 diabetes and better regulate their blood sugar levels.

7. Improved quality of life:

- Independence: Exercise improves functional strength and mobility, enabling women to age gracefully.
- It may alleviate chronic pain conditions such as lower back pain and arthritis.

8. Weight Loss Role

- Calorie Expenditure: When combined with a balanced diet, exercise helps to produce a calorie deficit, assisting in weight loss or maintenance.
- Strength training promotes lean muscle mass, which may increase resting metabolism.
- Exercise is essential in a woman's life since it benefits her physical health, mental well-being, emotional stability, and overall quality of life. To get the full benefits, participate in a variety of exercises tailored to individual objectives, fitness levels, and interests. Women with particular health difficulties or medical conditions should get advice from a healthcare provider or fitness consultant before commencing any new training routine.

Exercises to Reduce Metabolic Confusion.

Workouts for metabolic confusion are designed to keep your body guessing and adapting to different workout types, intensities, and durations. Here are some examples of exercises that employ metabolic confusion to boost your metabolism and help you achieve your fitness goals. To prevent injury, always warm up before exercising and cool down afterward.

HIIT Circuit: High Intensity Interval Training time: 20-30 minutes.

Preparation time: 5 minutes.

- Jack-knife leaps.
- Squats are performed with just your body weight.
- Arm motions.

Exercise for 20-25 minutes.

After 45 seconds of each exercise, allow 15 seconds for relaxation. Finish 3–4 rounds.

- Mountain climbers doing burpees
- Dumbbell or kettlebell swings.
- Push-ups
- With shoulder taps, perform a plank
- Squat jumps.
- Cycling crunches.

Refreshment (5 Minutes):

- The hamstrings, quadriceps, calves, chest, and shoulders should all be stretched.

2. Combining cardio with strength:

- in 45 minutes
- Warm up for 5 to 10 minutes.
- Jump rope or jog while stationary dynamic stretches: arm circles and leg swings.

Exercise Your Strength (20 Minutes)

- With a minute between sets, do three sets of 10-12 repetitions for each exercise.
- Squats with a barbell or dumbbell.
- Do dumbbell lunges, chest presses, or pushups.
- sagging rows

Holding a plank for 30 to 45 seconds, 15 minutes of aerobic intervals:

- Cardio for 30 seconds at strong effort, followed by 30 seconds of moderate recovery. Five times in a row.
- Tall knees.
- Jack-knife leaps.
- However, kicks fast skaters.

Refreshments (5 to 10 minutes):

- Static stretches: For major muscle groups, hold each stretch for 20-30 seconds.

3. Pyramid Exercise.

- 40 to 45 minutes.
- Warm up for 5 to 10 minutes.
- Arm circles and leg swings are dynamic stretches that may be done by jumping rope or walking fast.

Workout with a Pyramid (30 minutes):

- Begin each exercise with 10 repetitions, then lower the amount of repetitions by 2 every round until you reach 2.
- Hops while Squatting
- Push-ups, crunches, or sit-ups
- Dumbbell thrusters (using dumbbells of a medium weight)

Five-minute aerobic burst:

- Five rounds of 30 seconds of all-out effort and 30 seconds of recuperation should be accomplished.
- Running irregularly or on the treadmill
- Squat jumps.

Refreshments (5 to 10 minutes):

- Static stretches: Pay attention to the muscles you engaged throughout your exercise.

These sample workouts include high-intensity intervals, cardio, and strength training, all of which are critical to the notion of metabolic confusion. If you're new to training or have any underlying medical problems, see a fitness specialist or trainer, and remember to adjust the intensity and routines to your level of fitness. Always prioritize safety and pay attention to your body while exercising.

OVERCOMING CHALLENGES

Managing plateaus

Despite their frequency, fitness, and weight loss plateaus may be frustrating. When your progress stagnates despite your best efforts, a plateau forms. Making modifications to your workout and food regimen is required to properly cope with plateaus. The following are strategies for overcoming plateaus:

Change your exercise routine: Try new routines or modified versions of old ones. Changing your routine may promote development since your muscles adapt over time to the same movements.

- ***Increase Intensity:*** Gradually increase the intensity of your workouts by lifting heavier weights, doing more repetitions, or extending your cardio sessions.

- ***Incorporate HIIT:*** HIIT is a strategy that may be utilized to break plateaus. It fluctuates between brief rest periods and spurts of strong activity.

- ***Periodization:*** To decrease adaptation and increase progress, periodize your training by cycling through phases with different objectives (such as strength, endurance, and power).

Nutritional modifications: Track Your Food: Keep a detailed meal log to identify calorie traps and macronutrient imbalances.

- ***Calorie Adjustment:*** If you've been in a long-term calorie deficit, your body may have altered. Before returning to your deficit, consider temporarily increasing your caloric intake.
- ***Modifications to macronutrient ratios:*** Implement the required changes. For example, if you've been following a low-carb diet, consider gradually reintroducing healthful carbs.
- ***Meal Timing:*** Try various meal timings. Some individuals may find success by changing their eating habits or experimenting with intermittent fasting.

Recovery and Rest: Make Sleep a Priority. Insufficient sleep may limit development. Aim for 7-9 hours of quality sleep every night to help with healing and muscle development.

- ***Active Recovery:*** To minimize overtraining, alternate active recovery days with low-intensity activities such as swimming, yoga, or walking.

Stress Reduction: Cortisol Control: High stress levels might disrupt hormone balance and hinder weight loss. Practice stress-reduction techniques such as yoga, deep breathing, and meditation.

Professional Advice: Consider hiring a professional personal trainer who can assess your current routine and advise you on how to make beneficial changes.

- ***Registered dietician:*** A dietician can help you analyze your food plan and offer changes depending on your specific requirements.

Be Consistent and Patient: Remember that plateaus are an anticipated part of the journey. Keep your objectives in mind and try not to get discouraged.

Establish non-scale goals: Focus on accomplishments other than weight reduction, such as greater strength, endurance, flexibility, or a lower body size. These might help you remain motivated when you face a roadblock.

Reconsider Your Objectives: Think about your long-term goals. Are they still feasible and realistic? If required, adjust them to reflect your actual position and priorities.

Stay Hydrated: Sometimes a plateau is mistaken for dehydration. Make sure you receive enough water every day.

Think About Supplements: Consult your doctor before taking any supplements; nonetheless, some individuals may benefit from branched-chain amino acids (BCAAs) or creatine.

Maintaining Motivation

It may be challenging to remain motivated on your fitness journey, but with the right strategies, you can maintain your enthusiasm and achieve your goals. Here are a few tips to keep you motivated:

- **Set specific and achievable goals:** Set specific, quantitative, and reachable fitness goals. Having a clear aim to strive toward may assist improve motivation.

- **Create a Vision Board:** Create a vision board with photographs, statements, and reminders of your goals to help you envision them. Place it where you'll see it every day.

- **Discover Your "Why":** Determine the primary motivations for your fitness journey. Knowing your "why" may be a tremendous motivator, whether it's better health, more confidence, or setting a good example for your loved ones.

- **Break down your objectives into smaller steps:** Break down larger ambitions into smaller, more manageable milestones. To keep motivated, recognize your achievements along the road.

- **Establish a Routine:** Plan and adhere to a consistent training regimen. It will become a habit over time, making it easier to maintain motivation.

- **Change Up Your Workouts:** Workouts are more entertaining when they are diverse. To combat boredom, try out different exercises, courses, or activities.

- **Find a Workout Partner or a Community**: Working out with a friend or joining a fitness club may make it more enjoyable and accountable.

- **Reward Yourself:** When you reach certain goals, treat yourself. Non-food incentives may include acquiring new workout equipment or scheduling a massage.

- **Keep an exercise log or use fitness apps** to measure your improvement. Seeing progress may help inspire you.

- **Concentrate on Small-Scale Victories:** Rather than concentrating just on the scale, think about how your body feels, how your clothes fit, and other non-scale achievements.

- **Educate Yourself:** Learn the benefits of exercise and nutrition and how they affect your health. Knowledge may inspire and motivate you.

- **Visualize Success:** Spend a few minutes every day envisioning yourself achieving your fitness goals. Visualization might help you maintain your commitment.

- **Use of Positive Self-Talk:** Positive affirmations should replace negative thoughts. Be gentle to yourself and recognize your successes.

- **Podcasts and music:** Create exercise playlists or listen to motivational podcasts to keep you engaged and focused while working out.

- **Hire a Personal Trainer or Coach:** Consider hiring a personal trainer or coach to help with motivation, accountability, and specialized training.

- **Take on New Challenges:** Sign up for 5K runs, obstacle courses, and fitness challenges. Event planning may provide a sense of purpose and drive.

- **Plateau Adaptation:** Accept plateaus as a normal part of the journey and focus on the process rather than the end goal.

- **Rest and recuperation:** Make sure you get adequate rest and recovery time. Overtraining may lead to burnout and a lack of desire.

- **Be Patient:** Understand that improvement is not always linear. Be patient and persistent, even when things seem slow.

- **Look for Inspiration:** Follow fitness influencers or role models on social media to get daily inspiration and motivation.

A Sustainable Way of Life.

A sustainable lifestyle seeks to reduce one's negative impact on the environment and society while simultaneously boosting one's well-being and happiness. It requires making intentional judgments that consider the long-term consequences of our actions and strive for a balance of personal and global needs. The following are key attitudes and techniques for living a more sustainable lifestyle:

- Reducing, reusing, and recycling: Use fewer things, reuse them, and recycle materials such as paper, glass, and plastic.

- Energy Conservation: Use energy-efficient appliances, LED lighting, and programmable thermostats to save on electricity and gas.

- Transportation Sustainability: Reduce greenhouse gas emissions and air pollution by using public transportation, carpooling, biking, or walking.

- Environmentally Friendly Food Options: Choose locally produced and organic foods to help local farmers while also reducing the carbon footprint of food transportation and synthetic pesticides.

- Reduce meat consumption: Eating more plant-based meals helps to reduce the environmental impact of meat production.

- Water Conservation: To minimize water use, repair leaks, install low-flow faucets and toilets, and use water-efficient landscaping techniques.

- Eco-Friendly Fashion: Purchase clothes made from sustainable materials, support ethical fashion companies, and minimize your use of rapid fashion.

- Accept minimalism by decluttering and purchasing goods that are both valuable and long-lasting.

- Renewable Energy: To reduce reliance on fossil fuels, consider installing solar panels or purchasing power from renewable sources.

CONCLUSION

Finally, adopting a sustainable lifestyle is more than just a duty to safeguard the environment; it is a purposeful commitment to our planet's health and the well-being of future generations. Throughout this book, we've looked at a variety of sustainable activities, including eco-friendly behaviors, responsible living choices, and ways to promote personal health and satisfaction. During our investigation, we discovered the complex interaction between individual well-being, ecological stewardship, and the larger social influence of our everyday behaviors.

Individuals have the power to make a good difference in the world via their daily choices and habits. We can all help to make the world a more sustainable place by reducing waste, saving resources, and promoting sustainable principles. Simultaneously, by adopting healthier habits and maintaining our emotional and mental balance, we improve our quality of life. This synergy demonstrates the intrinsic link between sustainability and human development.

Furthermore, sustainability is not a one-size-fits-all paradigm; rather, it is a dynamic journey tailored to each individual's circumstances, ethics, and goals. It enables us to align our decisions with our beliefs and goals, building a route that reflects our sense of purpose and passion.

In our joint quest for sustainability, we recognize the enormity of the issues and the complexities of the solutions. Nonetheless, the intricacy of the situation encourages us to work together and remain committed. It encourages us to educate ourselves, engage in substantial discussions, and fight for policies and practices that prioritize the health of our planet and the well-being of its people.

In this comprehensive approach to sustainability, we find inspiration, empowerment, and a deep understanding of our interdependence. We understand that our actions have repercussions across society, affecting others' decisions and developing a culture of caring and responsibility.

Finally, pursuing a sustainable lifestyle is a never-ending journey—an adventure in which every step, no matter how little, contributes to the development of our planet. It is a journey that inspires us to live deliberately, purposefully, and harmoniously with our natural surroundings. As we begin on this journey, remember that the decisions we make today will shape the planet we leave to future generations. May our dedication to sustainability serve as a guiding force in our lives, improving not just our own experiences but also the common environment in which we all live. Together, we have the power to create a more sustainable, prosperous, and peaceful future.

www.ingramcontent.com/pod-product-compliance
Lightning Source LLC
Chambersburg PA
CBHW061005260726
48661CB00005B/2067